To Life!

To Life!

Artimia Arian

iUniverse, Inc.
New York Lincoln Shanghai

To Life!

iUniverse books may be ordered through booksellers or by contacting:

iUniverse
2021 Pine Lake Road, Suite 100
Lincoln, NE 68512
www.iuniverse.com
1-800-Authors (1-800-288-4677)

ISBN: 0-595-34184-5

Printed in the United States of America

Dedication

I dedicate this book to all those special souls who are willing to take the responsibility of their health into their own hands. By incorporating the knowledge provided in this little booklet into your daily lives, you will regain the most precious gift-your health and happiness.

Diseases are imbalances in the body caused by toxicity and deficiency. By cleansing the body of toxins and providing it with all the nutrients it requires, the body will once again return to a state of balance, a state of health.

The natural path is a sure path; a path with no dangerous side effects. However it is a path that requires an abundance of patience, perseverance and discipline. It is the path of the awakening of consciousness, the path of evolution. It is the path that leads to Light (knowledge) and Life.

I wish you the best of luck on this wonderful journey upon which you are about to embark. It is a journey that will change your life positively in countless subtle and overt ways.

To Knowledge! To Life!
With so much love,
Artimia

Contents

Useful Kitchen Tips

To Disinfect—For every liter of water add the juice of 2 small lemons (or 1 large) and 1 tbs. of sea salt. Wash the vegetables well with tap water and then let them sit in this lemon-salt water for 15 minutes. They must not remain for longer than 15 minutes as they will absorb the salt and the leafy greens will wilt. If the water is saved and used for disinfecting after an hour or more, add more lemon.

To Sprout—Soak the seeds in a bowl of water overnight. Remove the water in the morning, using a large strainer. Place the seeds in a large plate or tray and cover them with a humid cloth. Wet the seeds and cloth twice a day, morning and night, using a strainer to remove the excess water always. The seeds must never be too wet but they must not be allowed to dry. Within 3–7 days (depending on the seeds) your sprouts will be ready. They are ready to eat once the first two green leaves appear. Mung and lentil sprouts can be eaten earlier if desired. Sprouts can be refrigerated in tuppers or plastic bags.

Healthy Substitutes

Salt is substituted with sea salt, tamari, soy sauce or miso. As they all contain a lot of salt, they should be used sparingly. Seaweeds such as kelp, dulse and Nori are the healthiest salt substitutes.

Sugar (white, brown, molasses, etc.) is replaced by pure raw honey. Do not use more than 1 tbs. a day. Natural sugars found in fruits are best.

Oil: Cold-pressed unrefined oils such as olive oil, sunflower, sesame or coconut oil are good substitutes for all oils and butter.

Refined foods such as white bread, white rice, white pasta, biscuits made with white flour, etc. must be replaced by whole wheat products such as brown rice, brown bread, corn tortillas.

Food Combining Guidelines

1. DO NOT MIX PROTEIN WITH CARBOHYDRATES.

Protein—All Flesh foods (red meat, chicken, fish); Dairy Products (milk, butter, yoghurt, cream); Eggs; Legumes (Beans, Lentils, Soy products such as tofu; Nuts and Seeds).

Carbohydrate—Grains (rice, oatmeal, wheat); Pastas; Bread and Tortilla; Avocado; Tubercules (potato, sweet potato).

2. BOTH PROTEIN AND CARBOHYDRATE MIX WELL WITH A RAW VEGETABLE SALAD AND WITH CORN TORTILLAS. Eat one carbohydrate and one protein with steamed vegetables, a raw vegetable salad and corn tortillas.

3. FRUIT MUST ALWAYS BE EATEN ALONE. CITRIC (ACID) FRUIT (orange, pineapple, mandarine, etc.) DOES NOT COMBINE WELL WITH SWEET FRUIT (banana, dried fruit, mamey, etc.)

How much time to wait after eating a meal before eating again ?

1. **Most fruits digest in 20–30 minutes.** Dried fruit, banana, melon, mamey and watermelon digest in 40 mins. to 1 hour.

2. **After a raw food meal, wait 2 hours**.

3. **After a well combined cooked and raw food meal, wait 3 hours.**

4. **After a poorly combined meal, or a meat meal, wait at least 8 hours.**

Recipes

Dressings

1. Blend: Avocado, basil (or any other herb), lemon, garlic, soy sauce or sea salt, olive oil, water.

2. Blend: (For 1 liter of dressing) 4 avocados, cilantro, 1 clove of garlic, onion, soy sauce, juice of 2 lemons, water, fresh chili (optional).

3. Blend: Avocadoes, vegetables of choice (tomatoes, red or green bell peppers, celery, cucumber, zucchini, chives, etc.), soy sauce, juice of lemons, herbs of choice (cilantro, parsley, basil, thyme, oregano, etc.)

4. Blend: (For 1 lt. of dressing) ¼ large onion, 1 tomato, 1 large carrot, 1 small chili serrano (optional), juice of 1 lemon, olive oil, water, soy sauce.

5. Blend: Tomatoes, carrots, red bell pepper, cilantro, garlic, onion, miso (or soy sauce), olive oil.

6. Blend: Vegetables of choice (tomatoes, celery, zucchini, carrots, cucumbers, bell peppers), herbs of choice, garlic, onion, olive oil, soy sauce, water.

7. Blend: Soaked nuts and seeds (almonds, pecans, hazel nuts, walnuts, sunflower seeds, sesame seeds, etc), lemon juice, soy sauce, water, olive oil, herb of choice (cilantro, parsley, basil, mint, oregano, thyme, marjoram, etc.), honey (optional), mustard (optional), garlic (optional). Can add vegetables of choice (red bell pepper, tomatoes, fresh chili).

8. Blend: Sesame seeds sprouted or lightly toasted, olive oil, soy sauce, lemon, water.

9. <u>Blend:</u> 2 tbs. tahini or soaked sesame seeds, a small piece of ginger, garlic, 1 tsp honey, lemon.

10. Blend: 2 tbs. miso (or soy sauce), 2 tbs. onion, 1 clove garlic, ½ cup lemon juice, ½ cup orange juice, ¼ cup oil, ¼ cup water.

Salads

1. <u>Green Salad:</u> Lots of green leaves (watercress, different lettuces, chard, spinach, purslane, arugula); different herbs (parsley, cilantro, basil, oregano); any raw vegetable (tomatoes, cucumbers, carrots, red and green bell peppers, jicama, onion, celery, radish, zucchini, mushrooms, etc.); sprouts (alfalfa, mung, lentil, sunflower seed, etc.)

2. <u>Nopal Salad:</u> Lightly boiled nopales, diced, mixed with diced onion, tomato, cilantro. Add olive oil and soy sauce.

3. <u>Sliced Tomato and Onion Rings:</u> Sliced tomato and onion. Can add green pepper and/or sliced cucumber. Add olive oil, lemon juice, soy sauce.

4. <u>Guacamole:</u> Mashed avocado mixed with diced chives and cilantro. Add soy sauce and lemon juice. Any of the following diced vegetables can be added to the guacamole: tomatoes, celery, red or green bell peppers, radish, cucumber. Any green leaves can be finely chopped and added: arugula, chard, spinach, watercress. Add other herbs of choice such as parsley. Can be rolled into a large lettuce or cabbage leaf, or into a nori sheet (seaweed). Can add alfalfa or other sprouts.

5. <u>Ceviche:</u> Diced mushrooms, onion, tomato, cilantro, fresh chili such as serrano or jalapeno (optional). Add lemon juice, olive oil, soy sauce.

6. <u>Taboule:</u> Finely diced jicama, diced onion or chives and tomatoes, fresh parsley and mint. Can add diced cucumbers, red and green bell peppers, watercress (or other green leaves), olives. Add olive oil, lemon, soy sauce.

7. <u>Jicama Salad:</u> Large cubed tomato, jicama, bell peppers, celery. Add finely chopped jalapeno (optional). Dressing: any nut-seed dressing.

8. <u>Finger Salad:</u> Sticks of jicama, cucumber, carrot, celery. Dressing: any avocado dressing or nut-seed dressing or chili dressing.

9. <u>Lentil Sprout Salad:</u> Lentil sprouts, celery, cilantro, tomato, green pepper, onion. Dressing: olive oil, lemon, soy sauce.

10. <u>Chili Salad:</u> Diced tomatoes, cucumber, bell peppers, radish. Dressing: lemon, soy sauce, cayenne pepper (or any other chili).

Soups

Cooked

1. <u>Cream of Broccoli (mushroom, chayote, carrot, etc.)</u> Steam the vegetables using clean water. When cooked blend the vegetables with the water used for steaming. Sauté garlic, onion, celery, parsley or any other vegetables or herbs in soy sauce and water (in a Teflon pan). Mix everything together. Part of the steamed vegetables or herbs can be blended, and part chopped up and mixed in afterwards. Soups can be blended with any soaked nuts or seeds such as almonds, pecan, sunflower seeds. Top soups with: cubed avocado, chopped parsley, oregano, basil, chives, arugula, cilantro, diced tomato, radish, onion, celery.

2. <u>Mixed Vegetable Soup.</u> Cut up any vegetables of choice e.g. chayote, calabasita, broccoli, cauliflower, zucchini, onion, tomatoes, mushrooms, etc. Boil in a pot of water. Add herbs and spices, and a salt substitute such as soy sauce. Alternatively can boil a pot of water and add any cut vegetables of choice, with herbs, soy sauce and chili (optional). Cover and allow to sit for 15 minutes. Can add sautéed onion, garlic, herbs. Can also blend tomatoes, onion, garlic, any other vegetables, herbs, and add to the soup.

3. <u>Quick Soup.</u> Blend hot water, soy sauce, olive oil (optional) with vegetables such as tomato, avocado, onion, garlic. Add grated or cut vegetables such as zucchini, carrots, celery, cauliflower, peas, green leaves. Add finely cut herbs.

Raw

1. <u>Vitality Soup</u>—Blend tomatoes (with no water), seaweed (nori, kelp), little soy sauce, lemon (optional), olive oil (optional). Add any other hard vegetables and herbs of choice and blend: celery, carrots, bell peppers, cucumbers, zucchini, radish, parsley, cilantro, basil. Top with cut greens, avocado, onion,

radish. Alternatively juice any vegetable juice in the extractor (carrot, red bell pepper, celery) and use this as the soup base. Add any grated vegetables, sprouts and greens.

2. Lentil Soup: Blend many tomatoes, 1 red bell pepper, cilantro, chives or onion, 1 or 2 sticks celery juice, a little carrot juice, jalapeno, soy sauce. Add chopped onion, tomato, cilantro, celery (optional). Mix all together and add lentil sprouts. Eat with greens such as arugula.

3. Gazpacho: (Serves 6) Blend 2 kg tomatoes, 2 red bell peppers, 1 green bell pepper, cilantro, garlic, 3 celery stalks, 2 cucumbers, ½ small onion, 2 lemons, soy sauce.

4. Avocado Soup: Blend 3 tomatoes, ½ cucumber, 1 stalk celery, ½ onion, 1 tbs. chopped parsley, 2 avocadoes, juice of 3 lemons, soy sauce. Top with sprouts.

5. Cream of Spinach Soup. Blend 2 cups tomato, celery and carrot juice, 2 cups spinach, ½ avocado, little garlic, 1 tbs. jalapeno, 1 tbs ginger (optional), 2 tbs. onion, 1 tbs. mint, ⅓ cup cilantro, juice of 1 lemon, olive oil, soy sauce.

6. Carrot Tomato Soup. 4 carrots, 3 tomatoes, a handful of almonds, a handful of arugula, soy sauce. Blend well. Add chopped cilantro.

7. Green Soup. ½ avocado, 1 tomato, water or coconut water, lots of greens, juice of ½ lemon, soy sauce.

8. Raw Veggie Soup. Blend 4 tomatoes, ½ red bell pepper, 1 cucumber, jalapeno to taste, soy sauce. Top with shredded greens (tapsoy, arugula, cilantro, etc), grated carrot, zucchini, radish, chives (and any other vegetable), cubed avocado.

Steamed Vegetable Dishes

Steam any vegetables whole, diced, sliced or grated. Cut vegetables must cook for less time. Most vegetables must be cooked for no longer than 5 minutes. Cook the harder vegetables such as carrot, chayote, broccoli and cauliflower first. When they are half done add the softer vegetables which cook faster such as zucchini, mushrooms, green beans. Top with soy sauce, lemon, oil or any dressing of choice. In a Teflon pan sauté onions, garlic and herbs of choice in soy sauce and water on a very low flame for 2 mins. Turn off and add oil. Add to steamed vegetables. Good vegetables to steam are: carrots, broccoli, cauliflower, cabbage, beets, zucchini, green beans, onions, aparagus, chayote, corn, mushrooms, eggplant, snow peas, brussel sprouts, artichoke, purslane or any other green (spinach, chard). Greens are steamed for less than 1 min.

Examples of Steamed Dishes

1. Steamed carrots, broccoli, asparagus, peas—mixed with sautéed onion.

2. Steamed green beans, chayote, cauliflower—mixed with sautéed onion.

3. Shredded cabbage, mung sprouts, celery, red and green pepper, carrot, broccoli—mixed with sautéed onion and mushroom.

4. Artichokes (steam for 40–60 mins) served with basil or other dressing.

5. Eggplant—peel and slice thinly. Steam. Blend: tomatoes, garlic, soy sauce. Cook everything in pan for 10–15 mins.

6. Green leaves such as purslane, chard or spinach—steam for less than 1 min. Serve with lemon, sea salt, kelp (optional), soy sauce, olive oil.

7. Chop Suey—sauté onion, green bell pepper and mushrooms in soy sauce for 1–2 mins. Cover. Add the following vegetables cut in thin strips and steamed: broccoli, jicama, carrot, zucchini, mung sprouts. Add olive oil.

8. Stir Fry. Steamed or dehydrated, and diced or sliced: onion, mushrooms, broccoli florets, zucchini (long thin strips), celery, red and green bell pepper, eggplant. Raw diced or long thin strips: carrots, jicama, mung sprouts, peas, beet, almonds (small pieces). Combine. Dressing: soy sauce, oil, orange juice.

Vegetable Juices

Green Drinks

Green drinks are one of the most nutritious foods and most powerful natural medicines. They make the body more alkaline. Most people have an acid body condition due to the consumption of acid-forming foods such as flesh foods, bread, tortillas, pasta, dairy products and all junk food. Negative emotions also produce more acids.

Green drinks nourish and reconstruct the cells and tissues of the body. They aid the elimination, assisting the body to expel toxins that have accumulated over the years.

Any green leafy vegetables can be juiced. Here are a few examples: spinach, chard, parsley, dandelion, watercress, arugula, kale, beet and carrot greens.

1. <u>Green Citric Drinks</u>. Blend any green leaves with water and strain. Add any citric juice such as orange, grapefruit, pineapple. Half citric juice and half greens and water.

2. <u>Greens and Celery Juice</u>. Start out with ¼ glass of greens juiced in the juice extractor (Green Life or Green Power are the best extractors for greens) and ¾ glass celery juice. Cucumber and lemon juice (or other citrics) can also be added. Slowly increase the amount of green juice and decrease the amount of celery juice.

3. <u>Greens and Apple Juice.</u> Greens also combine well with apple juice. Use the juice extractor. E.g. Juice: 4 apples, some parsley, a bunch of chard. Juice: 1 large apple, 5 celery stalks, 1 bunch parsley, 1 bunch spinach.

4. <u>Greens and Tomatoes and Cucumber Juice.</u> (Do not use if the body is too acidic). Juice: any leafy greens, 6 small tomatoes, 1 cucumber, 4 celery stalks (and leaves).

5. <u>Greens and Carrot Juice.</u> Any greens mixed with carrot or jicama juice.

Vegetable Drinks

1. <u>Spinach and Carrot Juice</u>. $1/3$ spinach and $2/3$ carrot juice.
Spinach is excellent for the stomach, small and large intestines. Spinach (and all green drinks) are extremely effective for constipation.

2. <u>Carrot, Beet and Cucumber.</u> $2/3$ carrot, $1/3$ cucumber and beet.
This juice is excellent for gravel or stones in the gall bladder and kidneys and for prostate and other sex glands problems. It is also good for rheumatic conditions. Parsley mixed with this juice is good for promoting menstrual discharge.

3. <u>Potassium Drink.</u> Little less than ½ carrot and little more than ½ spinach, parsley, celery. This is a complete nourishing food. It is also outstanding in reducing stomach acidity.

4. <u>Carrot and Celery</u> (½ of each). Good for rheumatism, arthritis, asthma and allergies. Also good for arthritis is grapefruit juice.

5. <u>Carrot and Cabbage.</u> ⅔ carrot and ⅓ cabbage. Good for cancer. Carrot and carrot and spinach are also good for cancer.

6. <u>Carrot, Celery and Apple.</u> Equal quantities of each. Good for diarrea.

7. <u>Carrot and Apple.</u> Equal quantities of each. Good for colitis.

8. <u>Carrot, Celery, Parsley.</u> Mostly ½ carrot and ½ celery, and a little parsley. Good for nervous disorders.

9. <u>Carrot and Beet.</u> ¾ carrot and ¼ beet. Good for tumors.

10. <u>Carrot, Beet and Celery</u>. ½ carrot, nearly ½ celery, a little beet. Slowly add more beet as the body tolerates it more. It is a great blood cell builder and is therefore excellent for anemia.

Special Properties of Juices

APPLE: Healer of intestinal inflammation, helps the digestion.
BEET: Cancer-tumor healer; blood builder.
CUCUMBER: Alkalinizer, mineralizer.
CABBAGE: Vitamin U; healer of ulcers.
CARROT: Best balanced in vitamins and minerals.
CELERY: Alkalinizer; good for the nervous system.
DANDELION: Alkalinizer; has a lot of magnesium which is important for the bones. Is a blood builder as has a lot of iron. Is a kidney and liver cleanser. Is a great tonic.
LEMON: Rich in bio-flavonoids.
PARSLEY: Helps glands, nerves, blood coagulation, eyes.
TOMATO: Fruit richest in minerals.
ORANGE: Rich in calcium, phosphorous, vitamins C and A.
WATERMELON: Alkalinizer, kidney activator and cleanser.

Breakfast Options

1. Citric (Acid) and Sub-Acid Fruit. Orange, grapefruit, lime, mandarine, pineapple, guava, grapes, kiwi, apricot, plum, blueberries, raspberries, strawberries. Can be eaten whole, in a fruit salad or blended, one or a combination of fruits.

Examples of Citric Fruit Purées. Blend the following:

Orange juice and water (½ juice ½ water)
Orange juice and pineapple
Orange juice and strawberries
Orange juice, pineapple, strawberries
Orange juice and guavas
Orange juice and peach or plum
Mandarine juice and water (½ juice ½ water)

Citric fruit combines well with nuts and seeds. Can eat a handful of soaked nuts and seeds with a citric fruit breakfast.

2. Melons. Watermelon, cantaloupe, sweet green melon. Melons must be eaten alone. Can be blended or eaten whole.

3. Fruit Salad. Cut up an assortment of fruit. Dress with blended almonds, banana and orange juice. Top with cinnamon.

4. Sweet Fruit Purées

Blend:
Banana, papaya, water
Banana, mango, water
Banana, dates, vanilla (optional), water
Apple and a little water
Zapote or mango and orange juice
Banana, strawberries, peach
Mango, raspberries, peach

5. Green Drinks

Pineapple, orange, spinach, lemon. Blend and strain.

Any green (comfrey, parsley, chaya) blended with water and strained and then added to apple or orange (mandarine, grapefruit) juice.

Daily Menu

UPON ARISING:

Drink the juice of 2 to 6 lemons in double the amount of water (or more), using a straw to protect the teeth.

BREAKFAST:

See Breakfast Options.

MID-MORNING:

1–2 lts. Green Juice and Vegetables.

LUNCH:

A large green salad or other raw food dish (70 % of the meal at least) and steamed vegetables or soup.

MID-AFTERNOON:

1–2 lts. Vegetable Juice.

DINNER:

As for lunch or fruit.

NIGHT: (After digestion is completed)

Fruit.

Therapies

1. Enema—You will need an enema bag or little plastic bucket which is sold with a long rubber tube extending from the enema bag or bucket to the plastic cannula which is inserted into the anus. You must also purchase a water-soluble lubricating gel (not Vaseline—Lubrizal in Mexico or K&Y Jelly in the USA are examples). All of this equipment is bought in a pharmacy.

Lie on your right side on a mat or towel in the bathroom, right next to the toilet. There are many positions you can assume—lying on your back with knees bent or on your knees on all fours are two examples. Use whichever position is most comfortable.

Fill the enema bucket with slightly warm or room temperature water, or with chamomile tea (manzanilla). Refer to the tea preparation below. Place the lubricating gel on the anus and on the tip of the cannula. Gently insert the cannula into the anus. With your left arm (if lying on your right side) lift the enema bucket, allowing the water to flow with the force of gravity into the colon.

Whenever you feel at all uncomfortable or you feel the urge to release the water, remove the cannula and sit on the toilet. There should never be any pain. Repeat the process until at least 2 lts. of water have entered the colon. One should relax as much as possible, breathing deeply, whilst the water is running into the colon, thus enabling more water to enter.

The best time to do an enema is in the morning or in the afternoon (about 4 pm).

Tea Preparation—Boil 2 lts. of water. Switch off. Place a handful of chamomile tea into the water. Keep the lid on for 15 mins. Strain it and allow it to cool before use.

2. Foot Bath Therapy—You will need 2 small tubs, one for boiling water, the other for ice cold water. You must have 3–4 trays of ice handy and a lidded pot full of boiling water. You will also need a jug for pouring the boiling water from the pot to the little tub.

Fill one tub with hot water, as hot as your hand can stand it, and another with cold water and one tray of ice. Place both feet in the hot water tub for 5 mins. Then place the feet in the cold water for 5 mins. The water should reach the ankles. This operation is repeated 3 times (½ hour in all), ending with cold water. Add boiling water and ice whenever needed.

This therapy should not be practiced by pregnant women.

3. Cold Water Friction—You will need 2–3 trays of ice which will be emptied into a small tub of cold water. You will also need a small towel or facecloth.

The small towel is immersed in the ice water, wrung out, and starting with the left foot, you use the wet towel to rub the entire body vigorously, in the following order:

Front. Front of the right foot up the right leg, up to the right shoulder. Left foot to the left shoulder. Genitals up to the neck.

Sides. Right side of right foot upwards, passing the right armpit, going down the right arm and then following up the right arm, ending at the right side of the neck. Repeat on the left side.

Back. Starting behind the neck, moving down the back, to the buttocks. Back of the right leg and under the right foot. Back of the left leg and under the left foot.

After each movement, the towel is returned to the cold water and wrung out. One wants the towel as cold as possible all the time.

After the cold water friction you can return to bed without drying yourself (place a dry towel on the bed and another over the body), or you can exercise, dressing without drying yourself. In either case you do not dry the skin. The idea is that the cold water friction does not provoke cold. The heat reaction immediately afterwards is important for its effectiveness and to prevent you from catching cold. Air currents should be avoided.

4. Cold Sitting Water Bath—You will need a bag of ice or 10 ice trays. Fill a tub with cold water to cover the waistline when seated. Sit in the tub with the knees and feet outside of the water. Begin with room temperature water, adding ice as the water warms. If you feel cold, you can place the feet in warm water or wear socks. You can also cover the upper part of the body. Another option is to place the tub in the sun and wear a bathing suit, or heat the bathroom with an electric heater.

Every 5 mins. add another ice tray. One can sit in the bath for as long as desired, but a suggested time is 40 mins. to 1 hour. The longer, the more effective.

Women should not practise this therapy whilst menstruating or pregnant.

Cosmic Medicine and Healing

The physical body is a whole and has different necessities, all of which must be met, for an individual to function optimally. The tendency in Allopathic Medicine and the different Alternative Medicines, has been to specialize and use only that specialization to heal the patient. We have to realize that we are composed of four components: a physical, emotional, mental and spiritual body. Health is a state of freedom existing on the four levels. A healthy person experiences physical vitality and freedom from physiological malfunction, emotional peace and freedom of expression, mental clarity with creativity, and spiritual freedom due to a strong God-connection, which guides his life, bestowing order, harmony, peace and happiness.

In a cure, all four vehicles have to be taken into account, or at best the cure will be temporary, or at worst it will not be effective at all. All the bodies are interrelated, each one affects and is affected by the others.

Many people today are using one-sided methods such as vitamins (or minerals or enzymes), massage, special diets, exercise plans, special herb teas, etc. None of these approaches is sufficient in itself. There is no universal "cure all." Healing must be holistic, taking into account the spiritual, mental, emotional and physical well-being of each person. The person's lifestyle must incorporate all these components.

In the physical body, we have to consider the following parts: chemical and structural/energetic. We can only achieve a chemical balance in the body by improving the blood chemistry principally through correct nutrition. Herbology and Homeopathy can contribute to the blood chemistry to an extent, although they are not limited to this aspect. However, through correct nutrition and taking into consideration the individual's vibration and the vibration required by the body at a certain period in time (this information must be received), and correlating this with laboratory tests (blood tests or hair analyses, etc.), one can correct the blood chemistry.

The structural/energetic body area is covered by any therapy which employs physical and energetic methods to correct the energetic flow of the patient, thus improving the blood circulation and improving the functioning of all the organs. Included in this category are all the physical therapies such as chiropractic, polarity, osteopathy. Also included would be Chinese acupuncture, massage, reflexology, Yoga and Tai Chi, Reiki and energy cures.

George Vithoulkas, a respected contemporary homeopath, has outlined the varying depths of symptoms from each level (1980; 24), in descending order of depth, symptoms and their impact on one's state of health.

Physical	*Emotional*	*Mental*
Brain ailments	Suicidal depression	Complete confusion
Heart ailments	Apathy	Destructive delirium
Endocrine ailments	Sadness	Paranoid ideas
Liver ailments	Anguish	Delusions
Lung ailments	Phobias	Lethargy
Kidney ailments	Anxiety	Dullness
Bone ailments	Irritability	Lack of concentration
Muscle ailments	Dissatisfaction	Forgetfulness
Skin ailments		Absentmindedness

The physical body is the grossest of the four bodies and is the easiest to heal, provided the person is disciplined enough to follow a personalized dietary regime, specific to his/her vibration and provided s/he is living the correct life experience corresponding to his/her chakra life lesson (Refer to Cosmic Reawakening by Artimia Arian).

The spiritual body, the subtlest of the bodies, is the most difficult to heal. Spiritual body problems manifest in the emotional body and are evident in deeply ingrained non-functional behavioral patterns. People who have attained Chakra 4 or above in a past life, must be dedicating their lives to service of humanity, for the health of their emotional bodies. The spiritual body can also affect the mental body in severe cases. The spiritual body can only be helped by the individual first working to heal all the other bodies, and then attempting to connect to the Higher Self, which will offer the necessary information for the healing of the spiritual body. If the person is not well connected in Chakra 6 (most people), it would be wise to get help from someone well connected.

Orthodox Medicine Versus Holistic Medicine

Both systems of medicine are valid and actually essential to modern day living, however one should know when to resort to Allopathic Medicine and when to utilize Natural Medicine.

Holistic Medicine encompasses a holistic natural way of life. "There are no sicknesses, there are only sick people," said Hippocrates. The only "sickness" that exists is "ignorance of health," and the only logical remedy is the instruction of the individual, teaching him to follow Nature's Laws, living a healthy life. In Holistic Medicine, the patient is taught correct nutrition and how to use the natural elements to recuperate his health, without the necessity of foreign, artificial interventions, which are considered harmful, such as medicines, surgery, etc. Holistic Medicine teaches a system of life, which cultivates health. If natural laws have been violated, one does not need to combat a sickness, one needs to re-establish and maintain integral health. Holistic Medicine acts upon normalizing the functioning of the organism, a positive phenomenon. Holistic Medicine treats the patient, not the disease.

Health is balance in the system. Disease is imbalance. According to Dr. Robert Young's research (Refer to his outstanding book, "Sick and Tired"), in an unbalanced environment, morbid bacteria can issue from our own healthy cells. These tiny life forms can rapidly change their form and function. Thus bacteria can change into yeast, yeast to fungus, fungus to mold, in a process he calls pleomorphism. Therefore, the condition of your terrain is all-important. Your terrain is considered to be the ecological environment of the body (the blood, body fluids, lymph and digestive tract). Instead of focusing on combating the wealth and diversity of symptoms, we must cleanse and balance our system. There are no enemies or specific diseases to fight. There is a system in balance or our of balance.

According to Dr. Robert Young (Ph.D., D.Sc. in Microbiology and Nutrition), who has devoted his life to research into the causes of "disease," negative thoughts, emotions and an acidic diet lead to the disorganization of cells and a resulting unbalanced environment. In such an environment, healthy cells change form and become unhealthy cells (germs which are bacteria, yeast/fungus and molds). We all know that there are germs everywhere, but if your inner terrain is clean and balanced, the germs could not propagate in your system and take control, resulting in the plethora of symptoms and "diseases." Dr. Robert Young is not alone in his research findings. His work is an extension of many doctors and scientists dating back to the 1800s. They all confirm the scientific doctrine of pleomorphism that Antoine Bechamp (1816–1908) introduced over one hundred years ago.

Allopathic Medicine, acts upon the sickness, a negative phenomenon. Allopathic Medicine is based upon the premises that we are victims of often mysterious, malignant and capricious microbes and infections that attack us. Allopathic Medicine focuses more on the disease than on the individual. It groups a list of symptoms into a disease name, in order to identify and administer the drug that will suppress those symptoms.

Both systems of medicine are valid, if used correctly. If we violate Nature's Laws we will suffer from toxic accumulations or mineral deficiencies, usually in the inherently weakest organs or tissues, manifesting as all the different pathological diseases prevalent today. Thus the natural healers are one hundred per cent correct in wanting to teach man first and foremost how to manage and care for his physical vehicle. Ignorance of the health laws has created and continues to create, so much unnecessary fear, suffering and premature deaths. There is no knowledge more valuable than the conservation of health if you have a physical body, because without this knowledge you are not be free to accomplish your work on Earth unhindered.

On the other hand, microbes do exist and man's physical resistance is frequently not optimal, due to weakened physical vehicles over the generations, and incorrect living habits. Microbes are always present in the body, but their percentage is usually low, if the internal terrain is balanced. If their percentage rises, due to man's toxic body, or low level of resistance, or any other reason, then problems arise. It is in these cases that drugs may be necessary. However, they should only be used in life-threatening situations, and as a last resort. Drugs and surgery have their place when properly used. The problem we are facing today is that they are resorted to far too frequently, compromising and weakening the inner terrain. Many operations could be avoided by proper diet and healthy living. Too often one operation follows another, because if one body part is missing, another is overburdened and eventually becomes exhausted. When drugs are used to suppress symptoms rather than correcting the source of the problem, they are being abused. When operations are used to try to excise weakened or toxic organs or tissues, rather than correcting the source of the problem, they are being abused.

Approximately 250 years ago there were no drugs or doctors using drugs. There were natural healers who all used natural remedies, exercise and correct mental outlooks to heal their patients. Hippocrates, known as the greatest healer the Earth has ever known, next to Christ, elected as the father of medicine by the medical profession, never used drugs. The Chinese were using natural healing methods 5,000 years ago, methods which we today are only beginning to use and understand, and then only the natural healers.

It is interesting to note that herbs, which were the only medicines at one time, are the forerunners of all drugs used today. Man isolated the active ingredient in herbs and manufactured it synthetically, enabling him to produce mass quantities at huge profits. However these synthetic drugs create many harmful side effects, contrary to their herbal counterparts, which are more effective and less expensive. The primary function of these synthetic drugs is to alleviate symptoms, not cure the root of the problem. Their herbal medicine derivatives, on the other hand, dispose of the symptoms by correcting the condition. Drugs, although effective in suppressing symptoms, weaken the body in the long run, lowering its level of resistance. Natural remedies, such as herbs or homeopathic remedies, restore normality without weakening the body.

Synthetic drugs have their place in emergency life-threatening situations, but they have been ineffective and should not be used on a day-to-day basis in the treatment of chronic diseases. Orthodox medicine is unsurpassed in treating acute infections and providing emergency treatments for accident injuries, where surgery is essential to reattach limbs or other equally impressive surgical feats. But drugs have been unsuccessful in the treatment of cancer, Aids, diabetes, heart diseases, and the long list of chronic pathological conditions. Medical records and high death rates in these conditions speak for themselves. Eighty percent of the diseases treated in the US are of a chronic nature.

The pendulum is once again swinging to the positive pole (natural healing methods, Chakra 6), as the Earth anchors more Cosmic Energy via individuals who are becoming more conscious (attaining Chakras 4 and above). With this renewed consciousness, natural lifestyles are adopted, and Allopathic Medicine will be used only for emergency treatments.

The higher one's vibration, the less capable the individual's physical body is of assimilating unnatural synthetic drugs. The higher your vibration, the more these drugs will damage your body. In Chakra 6 you will be guided from above not to ingest any form of medicine other than food, which you utilize as your medicine, to regulate your vibration, combating the sometimes uncomfortable effects of the Cosmic Energy.

Cosmic Life–Conscious Living

It is not death that a man should fear, but he should fear never beginning to live.
(Marcus Aurelius)

The environment you fashion out of your thoughts, your beliefs, your ideals,
your philosophy, is the only one you will ever live in.
(O.S. Marden)

Man lives his life in a maze and with blinkers blinding his vision; he is igno-rant as to how to live optimally whilst in the maze experience; ignorant that the maze experience is meant to terminate once he has lived all the essential pathways which lead to the maze exit. He therefore spends lifetimes living various pathways but never living others and not even realizing that he is meant to find the exit and then depart from the maze. He has no clear direction and no clear idea of what he is meant to achieve or where he is meant to be heading. He only knows to seek happiness and avoid pain and most of his growth evolves from this precept. He attempts to elect life alternatives which avoid pain, however he is not aware of his life lessons.

To exit the maze, one only has to focus on six life lessons and learn to live them correctly. These are the six chakra lessons.

Chakra 1, earn enough for money for yourself and your family, but have no excesses. The higher your consciousness, the less material possessions and pleasures will attract you, the more higher knowledge and pure love will attract you. Live as simply as possible in order to have the time and energy for higher pursuits. Simple living, high thinking.

Chakra 2, learn to relate harmoniously to a partner of the opposite sex, without losing your individuality, without either partner being co-dependent on the other. If Chakra 2 has been successfully lived, you will have no desire to relive the experience. As your vibration rises, your sexual desire diminishes, the Cosmic Energy becomes stronger and your greatest desire is service to humanity and your union with the Father. If you find a partner with these same desires (due to a vibrational affinity), then the two of you would continue together, but sex would not play a prominent role in the relationship, because of the elevated vibration of both partners.

Chakra 3, learn to master the food experience, knowing exactly what food the body requires (not what an undisciplined body or mind wants) at any given moment, and providing that food item. Strengthening the physical body through Chakras 1–6, so as to eventually leave the food experience. All chakra experiences are meant to be lived and left. Learning to be a balanced parent. Learning how to discipline with love. If your children seek your friendship and guidance once older, you were successful in your parenting role.

Chakra 4, embracing your spiritual team as your family. Becoming as close to your spiritual team as you are to your Earth family. Respecting your spiritual team even more than your Earth family perhaps, as their goals extend beyond one nuclear family, to the whole of humanity. Dedicating your whole life to your service, as part of this team, to humanity.

Chakra 5, wanting to share all the essential chakra life lesson knowledge you have acquired with others, knowing how much it has aided you on your path. Learning how to become an outstanding teacher, so as to impart this knowledge in the clearest way. Imparting all worthwhile knowledge you have acquired.

Chakra 6, learning to hear God and your Higher Self with clarity. Learning to trust your telepathy for your own guidance and to be able to guide your spiritual students.

Once these six life lessons have been completely mastered, you are ready to initiate your Cosmic Life Mission on Earth. This is the mission God has given you. By this stage you will be well aware of your Cosmic life above and you will know exactly what you will be expected to accomplish for God on Earth below. By living your life lessons consciously, you will have slowly been removing the blinkers marring your vision through the years, and by the time you attain the final stage of Chakra 6, your blinkers will have been removed. From here on fully conscious living is possible.

Cosmic living is conscious living and can only be achieved in a cosmic setting. In a Cosmic Ashram life, one has the opportunity of working Chakras

2–6 consciously. If your Chakra 1 has not been mastered, you may have to return to the world to work this chakra, as money does not really enter a cosmic lifestyle. If your were never able to earn a living, you should return to the world and learn this primary lesson, which cannot be learned in a cosmic world. If, however, you were successful in earning a living, but your Chakra 1 is not balanced, this could be worked in a cosmic world. If the chakra is too yin, meaning you are too tight with money, or too yang, meaning you are too great a spender, this will be rectified in your Chakra 4 group experience.

Cosmic living is conscious living and therefore entails an extremely intense living experience. The cosmic world cleanses peoples' past errors, not only from this lifetime but from all lifetimes. You zone in to the weakest body, which corresponds to certain life lessons, and this is what is mostly worked. You are well aware of where you are and where you are heading. Everyone in a cosmic world is heading for Chakra 6 and then Chakra 7. Every chakra experience is meant to be enjoyed fully; it isn't a race to end them as soon as possible. The more you put into each experience, the more you learn, and the better you are prepared for the one to follow. Each lesson builds on the previous one.

It is a very fast evolution in comparison to most people who frequently repeat certain chakra life lessons for many lifetimes, before they gain the consciousness to confront them rather than avoid them. It is only by confronting an unmastered lesson to which we have resistance, that it can be mastered. But because this path is such a direct one, leading you steadily to your goal, Chakra 6 and onward, your vibration should be constantly rising. As you surpass one obstacle and feel you have attained a comfortable plateau, you're moved on to the next lesson. It is therefore an intense living experience. Lessons that were learned in past lives are quickly relived in this life, depending on how fresh they are in your memory (which depends on how many lifetimes ago you lived the lesson.) A person who attained a high chakra in his past life, will move ahead move rapidly than a person who attained the same level but many lifetimes ago. The fact that he attained it many lifetimes ago, and not in his last lifetime, attests to the fact that he lost force (vision) in the interim between the lifetime he attained the high chakra and this lifetime. That force now has to be recuperated.

Cosmic living is all about focusing on fixing yourself, on recuperating lost force if you are an old soul, or gaining force if you are a new soul. This is an intense path because it is such a direct evolutionary experience. You evolve at an accelerated pace. However, everything must be viewed in a cosmic time frame. If there are only six life lessons you have to master in order to complete your human life experience (the aim of every birth on Earth), then do not consider five or ten years a long time to master a life lesson. An unlived life lesson usually takes approximately ten years to master. Any life lesson that has been lived, but not fully mastered, can take anything from one to ten years to master, depending on how much of it was mastered in a past life and how well you recall the lesson techniques (i.e. how many lifetimes ago you lived it). So although in a cosmic time frame ten years or twenty years is nothing, in Earth terms we see and feel this as a long long time.

One has to be totally committed to attaining Chakra 6, God union, in order to have the patience and perseverance to commit to and endure this exceptional path. Attaining Chakra 6 must be your only goal in life, your only desire, in order for you to achieve it, as all your energies have to be channeled in this direction. In reality, everyone ends up doing it anyway, most people just waste so much time and energy over it that a lot of unnecessary suffering is experienced before they become conscious. What has been created in Tashirat is a cosmic world on Earth, where people are given the opportunity of being guided through the chakra life lessons. Anyone who has taken a human body, must enter and complete the six chakra life lessons, there is no avoiding it. Procrastination (travel, amassing material gadgets, vacations, etc.) will only contribute to a loss of force, nothing more. Unconscious living is the norm; overliving a chakra experience to the exclusion of most other lessons. Our aim is to become completely whole people and for this to happen, we have to live all six life lessons fully.

Cosmic living burns all past karmas, it is a cleansing of the past through correct present actions (words mean little, only actions talk). Through your present actions you amend your past errors and thus regain force. You therefore undergo many curative crises on many levels (not just the physical), which aren't always comfortable or painless, but each one is a profound cleanse which is followed by a cleaner slate with which to reconstruct your life and with knowledge which provides direction so as to recuperate lost force. Force is lost when an individual attains Chakra 4, 5 or 6 in a lifetime (he dedicated his life to God) and then returns and gets stuck in a Chakra 1, 2 or 3 life experience. Travel or any other hedonistic living can be classified as a Chakra 1 experience. It requires money and you live for yourself. It is just one of the socially accepted addictions on Earth.

A cosmic lifestyle requires no restful vacations, as your life is paced in such a way that your daily life is more stimulating and enjoyable than any vacation could be. The money that would be spent on yearly vacations (most people spend a fortune on family holidays), is spent on improving your world, (a world for many), and therefore your life. Conscious, correct eating and living is difficult on a vacation, where you are surrounded by many worldly temptations. Isolated living close to nature in an Ashram-type environment is essential to help you ascend to Chakra 6. A protected spiritual environment is a necessity for the ascension of most people. Once you are well into the Chakra 7 life experience, you will have the strength to once again enter the world through your service. From Chakras 4–6, when the Kundalini Energy begins to diminish and the Cosmic Energy rises, one's service is performed within one's spiritual world.

There are many levels of consciousness and thus many corresponding worlds, but in the human life experience (Chakras 1–6), there are basically two broad categories of consciousness—a lower triangle Chakra 1, 2 or 3 consciousness and an upper triangle Chakra 4, 5 or 6 consciousness. There are many ways of viewing things and they are all correct, depending upon through which filter of consciousness you are seeing. Cosmic living corresponds to upper triangle consciousness.

Cosmic medicine and cosmic psychology differ enormously from all known fields of medicine or psychology on Earth, because they firstly take into account the level of consciousness of the person (what chakra the person attained in a past lifetime; how many lifetimes ago did s/he attain that chakra; what is the present state of his/her three bodies; how strong and how balanced each of his/her chakras are; which body is the weakest, thus the root cause of the problem; various other factors such as the person's vital force.) Once all of this has been established, one follows up with the more traditional diagnostic techniques and a healing program is designed.

Just as a program for a kindergarten child, a primary or high school child, or a university student, would differ enormously, according to their level of knowledge, so you treat your patients differently according to the knowledge they have accumulated over their lifetimes and according to their force, which is equivalent to their level of consciousness.

In the cosmic world, only Chakra 7 people are considered competent to heal others, meaning that only these individuals are able to guide others through the chakra life lessons, which they have already mastered. Healing entails mastering life lessons 1–6. What would happen if a Chakra 3 consciousness doctor tried to help a Chakra 6 consciousness individual who was undergoing a Cosmic Energy experience of which the doctor was totally ignorant (not having experienced it.) The diagnosis and treatment would be completely incorrect and would only cause confusion. The same would apply to a doctor of any level of consciousness that happened to be below the level of consciousness of the patient, regardless of how specialized and expert the doctor was in his field. He would be superb if the problem was a purely physical problem such as a broken bone. But many chronic physical problems (cancer, aids, diabetes, heart problems, etc.) have an underlying emotional or spiritual root that needs to be remediated in order to heal the condition.

Poems

Discipline

Where there is discipline, there is order.
Where there is order, there is harmony.
Where there is harmony, there is happiness.
Where there is happiness, there is force.
Where there is force, there is evolution.

My Dearly Beloved
(The Higher Self to the Human)

I am your Light,
I am your Life,
I am the Guide
By your side
Always.
Contact Me, Hear Me, See through My eyes,
In order to recognize Truth from false disguise.

I am your heart,
I am your pulse,
I am every breath you take.
When you're awake
You'll feel Me and hear Me constantly
Guiding you with My Light.
When your body is strong,
Your heart pure,
And your human mind is pushed aside,
You'll unite to Me and perceive
The Light in All.

Keep your vehicles balanced,
Body, emotions and mind,
So as to find
That peace of mind, that Bliss,
That magical kiss,
You exist!
And you are Me, you become the Light,
With all the knowledge, all the insight.
You are Pure Truth, Love and Light.

Hear Me, stay attuned to Me,
I am ever there,
Always near,
But you forget, confusing the manifestation for the Reality.
Look beyond the manifestation,
Look beyond all names and forms.
As you feel and hear Me within you,
Connect and feel and hear Me in the entire Cosmos too,
Guiding you...
With every whisper of the wind,
Every floating cloud
And bird twitter,
Allow the magical glitter of the Light
That permeates the Creation
To touch and connect you.

Never lose the connection, becoming a mere mechanical form,
A programmed robot.
Tune in to the Divinity
Of Creation, so as to Be
A form manifesting that Divinity,
Consistently, permanently,
Not intermittently,
In mere flashes.

I am you,
I am the True You.
Allow Me to express Myself,
Through you.

Connect to Me,
Permanently,
So together we can direct our vehicles,
Performing the task at hand perfectly.
As Creators we will construct,
Flowing with the Universal Seas of Energy,
Playing and creating Life.

My Dearly Beloved, Open to Me,
Permanently.
I am your Light,
I am your Life,
I am the Guide by your side,
Always.
My Dearly Beloved,
You are Me,
I am your very Self.
My Dearly Beloved,
I Am,
Always.
Purify, eliminate the negative in your human part so as to
Connect and Unite to Me,
Manifesting as the Divinity
You really are.

0-595-34184-5